Supplements for Women

Top 10 Fitness Supplements for Women

By: Bring On Fitness

© Copyright 2018 – Bring On Fitness – All Rights Reserved.

information contained within this document, including, but not limited to, errors, omissions, or inaccuracies.

About Bring On Fitness

Our passion for fitness gave life to **Bring On Fitness**. We started with the goal of helping as many people as we can. To educate, motivate and to help change peoples lives for the better. Bring On Fitness is not only for the fitness enthusiasts, but also for the beginner. We strongly believe nothing is more important than learning the basics and creating a strong foundation in both nutrition - through meal planning, and in exercise - by following a specific plan. This is just as important for the beginner, as it is for the experienced athlete.

We set high standards for ourselves, the information we share, and the products we carry. Our goal is to provide you with exceptional products that suit your needs and the knowledge and motivation to help you work towards and achieve your health and fitness goals.

Keep up to date by liking us on Facebook and Instagram @bringonfitness

And for a complete list of reads and a FREE GIFT check us out at: www.bringonfitness.com

"Our Mission is to have a positive impact in changing peoples lives. We will deliver the best possible fitness and nutrition solutions that will empower people to achieve their health and fitness goals."

Table of Contents

Introduction

I want to thank you for choosing this book, *"Supplement for Women: Top 10 Fitness Supplements for Women."*

What is the first thing that comes to your mind when you think of supplements? As far as women are concerned, supplements work as a good burning tool. But is that all? Most supplement marketing campaigns fail to get across the point, and we may not always realize this, but we need much more than a thermogenic fat burner. As women, we don't just wish to lose weight; we want to build a strong core and flaunt a fit body we can be proud of.

Today, a lot of women are interested in building muscle, flaunting abs, and building strength that can put men to shame. Of course, not everyone wants to build a body like a professional athlete, but most of us certainly wish to look toned and feel energetic.

To achieve a great body, just diet and exercise are not enough. Complementing your workout sessions with the regular consumption of supplements can make your body respond differently to the workout and diet plans.

If you are confused about which supplements you should take, we've got you covered with our strategic list of 10 best fitness supplements for women. We have put together a comprehensive list of supplements by explaining how exactly they can benefit you.

Regardless of whether you are a professional athlete trying to get a toned body or someone who simply wants to use supplements for health reasons, you will find this guide extremely beneficial.

I sincerely hope that you find the information provided in this guide helpful. Happy reading!

Whey protein

Most women shy away from using supplements, especially whey protein, owing to concerns that it will bulk them up. What women don't realize is that every woman's body is different, and consuming whey does not bulk them up. In fact, whey is an excellent source of protein and can help in weight loss.

According to several fitness experts, whey does not add bulk to women's bodies, as women don't have the hormone that promotes the development of beefed-up muscles in men. Rather, whey protein helps women to build a toned look rather than bulking them up.

How much whey should women consume?

The amount of whey to be consumed depends on the activity levels and how much the woman weighs. Most protein manufacturers recommend that women consume one scoop of whey once or twice a day, which is about 20 to 25 grams protein.

Do women need additional protein in their meals?

Women certainly need more protein than they get from their daily meals. Women who don't consume enough protein are at a greater health risk than those who eat ample amounts of protein on a regular basis. Some of the common health risks that they might face are:

- Edema
- Obesity
- Thinning of hair
- Fragile toenails and fingernails
- Increased risk of potential osteoporosis
- Slow metabolism

Reasons why women should be taking whey protein

- Whey protein is extremely easy to digest when consumed in liquid form or as a post-workout snack. It is also known to reduce cholesterol levels and body fat in women.
- Whey protein consists of essential amino acids like leucine, which can help to maintain lean muscle mass and promote fat reduction.
- Whey also contains glutathione, an important antioxidant that is required to keep a person's immune system healthy.
- Owing to a high content of essential amino acids and protein in whey, women can expect to build lean muscle, which leads to faster metabolism.

Creatine

What is Creatine?

Creatine is a natural compound that the human body produces; it converts into creatine phosphate within the body. It is known to be a great source of energy and helps to increase your stamina and promote faster muscle recovery in women.

Why is creatine important to women?

If you wish to strengthen your muscles and turn into a fat-burning machine without getting beefed up, creatine is the right supplement for you. You will feel stronger by improving the blood flow to your muscles, which results in effective contractions while you lift weights. It also provides your muscles with a constant supply of essential nutrients needed to shape your body.

Below are some reasons why every woman should take creatine.

Helps you nail your high-intensity workouts

When you lift heavy weights or run sprints, creatine can help you build endurance by maximizing your body's potential to produce energy. This happens because women who consume creatine can burn up to 70% of their phosphate stores within a span of 30 seconds with high-intensity exercise. Thus, when you have ingested enough creatine and head to the gym, you could be churning out greater lifts and faster sprints.

Helps you get better results

Have you been working out like crazy but can't seem to get the desired results? Creatine will help you achieve your fitness goals by fueling your muscles post workout, helping in the repletion of CP stores, aiding in muscle repair, and regulating better and faster workouts. Creatine may not change your body composition directly, but it will certainly help you by enhancing your high-intensity workouts, as well as your recovery from them. Regular consumption of creatine results in fat-free mass and a leaner physique.

Helps in a healthy pregnancy

Based on research, creatine can help promote healthy neural development while helping people recover from complications that arise out of inadequate oxygen supply. During pregnancy, a woman's body requires an increased supply of creatine as the fetus relies on the mother's creatine stores. Research shows that maternal creatine supplementation has been proven to help increase successful birth rates as well as organ function in animals. Several human studies have also proven that creatine supplementation can have a positive impact on fetal growth, health, and neural development during pregnancy.

Improves your mood

Although the exact mechanism behind this is not known, creatine can aid in alleviating symptoms of depression. One of the potential reasons for this could be the fact that creatine acts on neurotransmitter functions and balance in the brain.

Fish Oil

Most women think of "fat" as something to be feared, especially when they are trying to slip into new clothes. And it's not just the fat on the body; they seem to dread dietary fats, too. Omega-3 fatty acids like fish oil consist of poly-saturated fats that are required for optimal health. Given that the human body cannot produce omega-3 acids on its own, it is important that women consume fish oil supplements regularly.

One of the biggest benefits of taking fish oil supplements is that it aids in better heart health. Fish oil helps to reduce blood pressure levels, regulates heart rhythm, slows down the clogging of arteries, and lowers blood fat levels. Aside from these, there are a few other advantages of regular consumption of fish oil.

Below are some reasons why women should take fish oil supplements.

Helps ease menstrual pain

Many women endure extreme abdominal discomfort during those days of the month, mainly due to a condition known as dysmenorrhea. It is caused by the intense contractions of the uterus as a result of prostaglandins (chemicals that are linked to inflammation and pain). Based on studies, women who consume omega-3 on a regular basis experience a reduction in menstrual pain. It is also helpful in stabilizing your mood and getting your hormonal fluctuations under control.

Alleviates the symptoms of rheumatoid arthritis

Rheumatoid arthritis impacts women more than men. Some women suffer from severe symptoms that make it difficult to carry on with their daily lives. Several researchers have shown that fish oil supplementation can significantly reduce stiffness and joint pains in patients who have rheumatoid arthritis. That being said, don't stop taking medications that are prescribed by your doctor while you consider fish oil supplements for your arthritis symptoms.

Protects against osteoporosis

Osteoporosis occurs because of the loss of bone density as a person starts to grow older. Owing to lower bone density, women are obviously at a higher risk of developing osteoporosis as compared to men. Women who have a genetic predisposition are at an even higher risk. A review linking omega-3 and osteoporosis published in 2012 in the British Journal of Nutrition shows significantly favorable results of omega-3 on patients' bone density.

Keeps your mood elevated

Fish oil supplements are also known to be a great mood enhancer. Some recent reviews have also found that fish oil supplements can be greatly effective against depression. Although the evidence isn't very strong, a lot of women have experienced a sudden positive change in their mood after taking fish oil supplements. Many researchers are of the opinion that more controlled studies need to be conducted in order to determine the long-term benefits of using fish oil to treat depression.

Keeps your skin clear and hair shiny

Fish oil can do wonders for women's skin and hair. It keeps the skin hydrated and keeps it soft while helping in the production of healthier skin cells. It can also make your hair stronger and shinier while keeping your scalp healthy. Fish oil has also been linked to improvement in wrinkles and psoriasis. The Mediterranean diet, which is high in omega-3 oils, has also been proven effective in treating acne in women.

Casein

Protein plays a significant role in nutrition, as it helps in the proper functioning of the body, strengthens it, helps build muscle and also aids in recovery post workout. That being said, not all protein gives you the same results. Men, as well as women, use casein to help develop lean muscle mass in conjunction with their daily workouts. Aside from the fact that casein and whey are derived from milk, they are completely different from each other. Casein protein makes up about 80% of milk as compared with whey and offers several benefits.

Below are some reasons why women should take casein.

Slows digestion

Since casein molecules are bigger than whey molecules, they are easily digested and get absorbed slower. Drinking whey protein can spike up your blood amino levels, and while it gets absorbed rapidly, this effect is short-lived. It also leads to slower digestion, making your body stay in the anabolic state for longer periods of time. Casein, on the other hand, works differently. A lot of people prefer to drink casein just before they sleep, so their body remains in the anabolic state while keeping the muscle mass at optimal levels.

Ensures rapid Success in muscle building

If you want to see faster results, casein protein is the way to go. For even better results, try using a combination of casein and whey together. Based on a 10-week study, when these two proteins are taken together, there is an increase in lean muscle mass, giving you toned legs and a shapely bum. Casein, when taken alone, can also be of great benefit for weight loss.

Enhances fat loss

If your aim is to lose the maximum amount of body fat, you should be consuming casein protein on a regular basis. Based on several studies, casein protein has helped both men and women lose fat faster. It happens because your body remains in a higher metabolic state longer after ingesting casein. This also helps you shed more fat as it takes a long time to digest, making you feel satiated for longer periods, due to which you are less likely to overeat.

Helps with great teeth

What makes you cringe more – your dentist's face or the dental chair? If you hate going to the dentist and want to maintain your dental health, adding protein to your diet can be the solution you are looking for. Research has found that casein protein is capable of preventing or reducing the impact of enamel erosion. If you have a habit of consuming a lot of fizzy drinks, which can rapidly erode your teeth enamel by the way, adding a bit of casein protein to your diet can save your teeth.

Improves colon health

Casein protein is highly effective in promoting colon health. The benefits of casein protein are reportedly higher than those of soy and meat. People who consume casein have reportedly experienced smoother bowel movements.

BCAA

BCAAs, also known as "Brain Chain Amino Acids," are the powerhouse aminos required to build muscle mass and accelerate the recovery process. The aminos that make up BCAAs are as follows:

- Valine
- Leucine
- Isoleucine

These are considered to be essential amino acids that the human body cannot produce. The amino acids that are regarded as extremely vital for the human body are tryptophan, valine, phenylalanine, threonine, leucine, lysine, isoleucine, methionine, and histidine.

Below are some reasons why women should take BCAA supplements.

Improves protein synthesis

BCAAs can trigger protein synthesis in the body, which allows it to be in the anabolic state for a longer duration. When you add high-intensity resistance training to a daily dose of BCAAs, the process of muscle tissue breakdown and recovery improves greatly. It's easier to tear down the muscles in the gym, but it's the recovery that is more important. BCAAs are valuable not only for muscle recovery from gym workouts but also for life in general.

Boosts immune system

Each time you train, you are exhausting yourself, leaving you at the mercy of your body's immune system. If your immune system isn't strong, you will start experiencing fatigue and chronic illnesses and eventually injure yourself at the gym. To get stronger, you need a healthier immune system to handle all the stress you are putting yourself through, and BCAA supplements can help you significantly. BCAAs can ensure that your energy levels are maintained and you don't become a victim of chronic stress.

Supports fat loss

Like most other supplements mentioned in this book, BCAAs can also help burn fat. Several surveys have shown that people who consume BCAAs in their daily diets have more muscle, less body fat, and better body composition. Based on a study conducted on 4,429 subjects, it was found that people with regular BCAA intake appear the slimmest and had a considerably lower chance of putting on excess pounds than people who don't consume BCAA.

Improves power

When you train, you don't do it just to maintain your muscle but also to enhance your body's power. Your goal should always be to stress your body, recover, and come back even stronger. Recently conducted training studies have shown that BCAA supplementation leads to a significant increase in leg press stress in gymmers. The reviews often mention a variety of protein supplementation responsible for this improvement, but all in all, BCAAs are considered to be rich in all the amino acids required for the body to recover and strengthen itself during the recovery period.

Reduces DOMs (Delayed Onset Muscle Soreness)

I am sure you know how difficult it feels to climb even a few steps the day after your leg day. Well, the soreness can be considerably reduced by BCAA intake pre and post workout. Most people assume that soreness is good for their body, but what they should be aiming for is minimal soreness, not the "can't even climb two steps" soreness. The sorer you get, the more you require a supplement that helps you with the recovery period, and BCAAs are excellent for that.

L-Arginine

L-Arginine is a non-essential amino acid, but there are times that the human body is not capable of producing enough, like if you are sick. Additionally, the amount of arginine produced by your body depends on gender, age, lifestyle, and drinking and smoking habits. Infants are unable to produce this amino acid in ample amounts, and its production only decreases with age.

Arginine supplements are the need of the hour, especially for women. It offers numerous benefits such as improvement in hair, skin, and health conditions. Arginine is also used to encourage female fertility as well as libido. Many women have also experienced a great improvement in their sexual arousal after consuming arginine as it increases blood circulation to the genitals.

Below are a few reasons why women should take arginine supplements.

Has anti-aging properties

As we all know, the human skin is the largest organ in the body, which loses its suppleness and elasticity with age. Regular intake of this amino through supplementation can sustain the vitality and beauty of the skin. Arginine is considered to be an HGH (Human Growth Hormone) enhancer, which helps to slow down the aging process. You don't have to spend a fortune on buying anti-aging products anymore. All you have to do is pop an arginine pill as per instructions, and watch your skin rejuvenate itself.

Promotes the healing of wounds

Arginine is known to promote the healing of wounds. Protein is vital for wound healing, and arginine helps to produce this compound, thereby making the recovery process faster. Many diabetes patients find it difficult for their wounds to heal. In such cases, arginine can help to shorten the recovery time for wounds, but it is advisable to consult a physician before you consume it. Arginine helps in the formation of L-proline, an essential compound for the formation of collagen to aid in faster wound recovery.

Repairs skin

If you have been struggling to get rid of acne, pimples, or scars on your face or hands, arginine can help to fix the damage. In fact, there are several skin care products in the market that contain arginine and are known to be super effective in fixing any type of skin issue. Arginine is also known to have antibacterial compounds, which, along with the anti-oxidizing agents, are capable of restoring skin damaged by environmental factors, such as dust or allergies. It can also help slow down the aging process while helping you restore youthful looks.

Stops hair fall

Arginine doesn't only stop hair fall but also promotes fuller hair. Arginine, an amino acid produced by the human body, can relax the blood vessels while enhancing blood flow to the scalp as well as the base of hair follicles. There are several benefits to add arginine to your daily hair-care routine including making your hair feel fuller, improving scalp health, strengthening the hair follicles, and promoting hair growth.

Prevents hair damage

If you like to color your hair often, you know what we are talking about here. Colored hair often goes through a lot of damage, leaving it dry, lifeless, and thin. To add to the misery, if you regularly step out in the sun, it only further damages the hair. Arginine can protect hair from heat and harmful chemicals. Owing to the fact that arginine can repair damaged hair, it is also used as a major component in most hair coloring products.

Beta Alanine

Beta alanine is an improved version of the amino acid called alanine. When consumed, beta alanine is transformed into dipeptide carnosine. Carnosine, which is stored in the body, acts as a trigger to buffer acid (pH) in case of intense physical activity. It can be stored in the muscle cells until the need arises, i.e., when the pH levels in the body go down. Beta alanine also helps you to train harder and for longer periods of time by protecting your muscles from experiencing fatigue as quickly as they generally do. Several researchers have studied the positive impact of beta alanine for years. These studies have also shown that the most recommended dosage for a significant impact is between 2 and 5 grams. The best thing about this supplement is that vegetarian as well as vegan dieters can consume it.

Below are some reasons why women should take alanine supplements.

Increases carnosine levels

Our bodies need adequate amounts of carnosine stores for proper functioning. It plays a vital role in the development of several organs, such as the liver, brain, heart, and kidneys. Carnosine is released when the human brain starts perceiving acidic body states, such as with lactic acid production during exercise. Carnosine is also known to act as an anti-aging agent and is used to treat type 2 diabetes mellitus.

Increases exercise capacity

A study conducted in 2009 and published in the Journal of Medicine and Science in Sports and Exercise showed that alanine can enhance muscle carnosine content and, therefore, has the ability to enhance physical performance during intense workout sessions. Some researchers have also found that certain aspects of endurance performance, such as anaerobic threshold and time to exhaustion, can be improved.

Benefits vegetarians

Meats are the best source of beta alanine and carnosine. Pork, fish, beef, and fowl are all loaded with this amino acid. Unfortunately, vegetarians may develop carnisine and beta alanine deficiencies. Many health care professionals recommend taking a daily dose of 4 to 5 grams of alanine supplements every day. If the dosage seems intolerable, you can divide it into smaller portions. It should be consumed at least two hours apart.

Boosts athletic performance

Based on human research conducted on beta alanine advantages, the following improvements in an athlete's performance were shown:

- Boost in power output during a sprint
- Boost in fatigue threshold
- Boost in total number of reps

- Improvement in ventilatory threshold
- Improvement in time to exhaustion
- Improvement in strength during bench press
- In a four-week study of beta alanine, a significant increase in endurance performance in runners was noted.

CLA

CLA is a fatty acid that is naturally found in dairy products from goats, cows, and sheep and in grass-fed meat. In the past few years, the positive impacts of consuming good quality fats have been highly researched, which has also shed light on several health benefits. CLA can be classified as one of those good quality fats and can be just what you need to explore your desired fat loss potential. However, even if you like indulging in dairy and meat, you may not necessarily get enough CLA from your food. The only way you can get enough of it is by eating tons of food until your stomach hurts, but who wants that? The best way to experience the advantages of CLA would be to take CLA supplements. If you are a woman, CLA supplementation can help you get the best out of your fitness schedule and nutrition while optimizing your body's fat burning capacity to get you closer to your desired goals.

Below are a few reasons why women should take CLA supplements.

Prevents cancer

CLA can protect the human body against cancer formation and progression. According to the National Academy of Sciences and Cornell University, CLA is the only fatty acid that can inhibit carcinogenesis among experimental animals. For this reason, CLA is considered to be effective in exerting an anti-cancer effect by promoting the body's capacity to absorb fat-soluble vitamins like vitamins A and D. This is done through the regulation of the growth and production of new cells and through its impact on prostaglandins, which are chemicals that regulate cellular function.

Prevents heart disease

CLA encourages the body to use stored fats as energy, which helps in preventing and treating certain kinds of heart diseases like atherosclerosis. According to the Pennington Biomedical Research Center, CLA helps in the prevention of plaque and lipid disposition in arteries, which is an essential factor in the growth and progression of heart diseases in humans. CLA can also act as an antioxidant agent and can lower blood pressure levels, thereby preventing heart disease.

Promotes fat loss

According to Pennington Biomedical Research, CLA helps in using body fat as the main source of energy, and this leads to a decrease in body fat levels in humans. CLA also helps boost the metabolic rate. Therefore, the advantages of CLA for fat loss can be considered a twofold process: by enhancing the metabolism of body fat while preventing the metabolic rate from slowing down while you are on a diet.

Multivitamins

Do women actually need multivitamin supplements? Today, there is considerable scientific data suggesting that a multivitamin supplement isn't all that necessary, but it's difficult to overlook the numerous benefits women have derived from it over the years. It is a well-known fact that people who ingest multivitamin pills on a regular basis are considered to be some of the healthiest on the planet. Many researchers have also concluded that vitamin takers turn out to be leaner, more educated, and more affluent people. A typical multivitamin supplement consists of up to 25 isolated nutrients, which can ensure good health. Most women today still need some strategic supplementation to make up for their dietary gaps. Some of the best multivitamins recommended for women are given below.

Vitamins A, C, and E

Vitamins A, C, and E are fat-soluble antioxidants that can fight against free radical damage, which is the reason behind several heart diseases and aging. Vitamin C is known to enhance your body's immunity against common cold, infections, or other illnesses. It also protects your skin against damage caused by UV light and environmental pollution. Vitamins A and E also work in similar ways to halt cell mutations and protect healthy cells, among several other benefits.

Vitamin D

Vitamin D can be easily obtained from food, such as dairy products, eggs, and certain types of mushrooms, but the major source of vitamin D is the sun. If your lifestyle requires you to stay indoors for extended periods of time, you are likely to develop a vitamin D deficiency. Some studies show that up to 75% of adults in the United States suffer from vitamin D deficiency. Vitamin D is also vital for brain functions, bone/skeletal health, hormonal balance, and mood regulation.

Vitamin K

Vitamin K is essential for the development and maintenance of strong bones. It prevents heart disease and blood clotting. Several women fall short of the required levels of vitamin K in their bodies, which puts them at a higher risk for cardiovascular diseases. Vitamin K is also helpful in alleviating the symptoms of inflammatory bowel disease or cholesterol issues. It is divided into two different types, namely, Vitamin K1 and Vitamin K2. Vitamin K1 is found in different vegetables, whereas K2 is found in dairy products.

B Vitamins

B vitamins, which include vitamin B12, are extremely important for boosting a woman's metabolism and cognitive functions and for preventing fatigue. Similarly, folate, which is among the B vitamins, is crucial for a healthy pregnancy, prevention of birth defects in baby's spinal cord and brain, and development of the fetus. Therefore, folate deficiency is considered to be fatal for pregnant women.

Caffeine Supplement

Whether you like the smell of caffeine or simply love the burst of energy it gives you, chances are that you don't know much about its extended benefits. Most of us look at our morning cup of coffee as a way of getting our day started, but there's much more to it. You can also take caffeine supplements for higher energy levels, better workout performance, and better brain function.

That being said, if you haven't consumed a caffeine supplement before or your body has a lower tolerance level for it, you should go slowly with its dosage. The recommended intake of caffeine supplements is between 200 and 400 milligrams. You can take these supplements one hour before and after workouts. If your body starts reacting adversely to these supplements with nervousness, heart palpitations, shivers, or anxiety, it's possible that you have overdosed on your caffeine supplements. Therefore, it is crucial that you take baby steps towards adding it to your daily routine and then work your way up.

Below are a few reasons why women should take caffeine supplements.

Provides an instant boost in energy

We all know how jumpy we feel after having a strong cup of coffee, but its effects on our energy go far beyond our knowledge. Pre-workout caffeine supplementation can improve poor training performance owing to sleep deprivation and boost our dopamine levels resulting in increased time to exhaustion. Many studies have shown that sleep-deprived people who take caffeine are able to perform as well as the ones who are well rested.

Decreases pain

According to a study published in The Journal of Strength and Conditioning Research, athletes who consumed caffeine prior to their resistance training experienced an immediate decline in their post-workout pain. The athletes also experienced a significant reduction in delayed-onset muscle soreness post training.

Aids in faster recovery

According to the Journal of Applied Psychology, when you combine caffeine supplementation with intake of fast sugars, such as dextrose, it can result in 66% higher glycogen repletion than when ingesting carbs alone. In fact, participants who consumed caffeine along with carbohydrates showed higher levels of blood glucose and a rise in their insulin levels, signaling anabolic drive. In order to accomplish faster recovery post workout, it is recommended that you ingest caffeine without adding any type of carbohydrates.

Other benefits of caffeine

- Reduces headaches
- Reduces constipation
- Sharpens mental focus
- Enhances memory
- Reduces pain perception
- Improves athletic performance

Conclusion

I wish to thank you once again for purchasing his book.

Remember that supplementation isn't food; so while you are trying to strive for a great body through supplements, don't forget to eat some real food, too. There are so many myths floating around the Internet trying to deter women from trying out supplements that I thought I had to come up with a book that offers some real facts about women's supplements. This book is a humble attempt to encourage women to take their health seriously and to stop them from fearing supplements just because someone told them that they would look like a man because of the bulk.

I hope this book has cleared most of your misconceptions surrounding women's supplements while encouraging you to add them to your everyday routine.

Thank you, and remember to share how well these Supplements for Women tips work for you. You can do that by writing a review in your Amazon account under Your Orders.

Thank you,

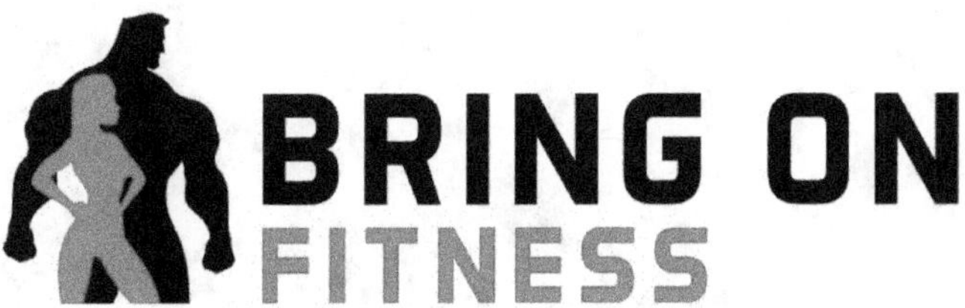

Resources

https://nootriment.com/beta-alanine-benefits/

https://www.mrvitamins.com.au/news/vitamins-minerals/5-reasons-womens-multivitamins/

http://womenwholiftweights.com/top-5-benefits-of-bcaas-for-women/

https://www.naturalstacks.com/blogs/news/creatine-benefits

https://www.webmd.com/vitamins/ai/ingredientmono-993/fish-oil

About Bring On Fitness

Our passion for fitness gave life to **Bring On Fitness**. We started with the goal of helping as many people as we can. To educate, motivate and to help change peoples lives for the better. Bring On Fitness is not only for the fitness enthusiasts, but also for the beginner. We strongly believe nothing is more important than learning the basics and creating a strong foundation in both nutrition - through meal planning, and in exercise - by following a specific plan. This is just as important for the beginner, as it is for the experienced athlete.

We set high standards for ourselves, the information we share, and the products we carry. Our goal is to provide you with exceptional products that suit your needs and the knowledge and motivation to help you work towards and achieve your health and fitness goals.

Keep up to date by liking us on Facebook and Instagram @bringonfitness

And for a complete list of reads and a FREE GIFT check us out at: www.bringonfitness.com

"Our Mission is to have a positive impact in changing peoples lives. We will deliver the best possible fitness and nutrition solutions that will empower people to achieve their health and fitness goals."